KIDNEY D
COOKBOOK FOR STAGE 3

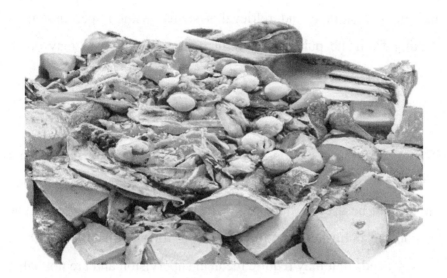

Tasty Recipes and Meal Plan To Manage CKD Stage 3 For Healthy Living

MICHELLE GREEN

FREE EMAIL CONSULTATION

Dear Reader,

Thank you for purchasing my book. As a token of my appreciation, I would like to offer you a free email consultation to help you clarify any concern in this book to your specific situation.

I understand that sometimes reading a book can raise questions or concerns, and you may be unsure about how to proceed. That's why I am here to help.

To take advantage of this offer, simply send me an email at michellediets101@gmail.com with the subject line "Book Consultation" and provide a brief description of the issue you would like to discuss. I will do my best to respond within 24 hours with actionable advice that will help you achieve your goals.

Please note that this offer is only available to readers who have purchased a copy of my book.

Thank you again for choosing to purchase my book, and I look forward to hearing from you soon.

MY OTHER BOOKS

I have other books that you could find helpful. Kindly scan the code below to gain access.

OR

https://www.amazon.com/author/michgreen

CONTENTS

INTRODUCTION

Stage 3 Chronic Kidney Disease (CKD) is a silent protagonist in the realm of health, a powerful force that frequently goes unrecognized until it's too late. Imagine for a moment Cynthia, my cousin's girlfriend. She appeared to be healthy, lively, and full of life, but beneath the surface, this sneaky disease was slowly killing her.

Cynthia was completely unaware that her kidneys were engaged in an epic struggle inside of her body. The dynamos that filter waste and maintain a delicate balance in place were failing. The gravity of her predicament only became apparent when she eventually learned that she had reached Stage 3 CKD. A severe sensation of despair developed from the initial shock, which then transformed into worry. Cynthia believed that all hope had been lost and that her ambitions and aspirations were vanishing with each dwindling heartbeat.

However, destiny had other plans for Cynthia, plans that would give her hope in the form of a fortuitous encounter. My cousin brought her to me and complained bitterly about how his girlfriend was becoming a shadow of herself. This situation was not new to me because I meet with such situations day to day as a dietitian. So, I offered assistance because I had witnessed Cynthia's struggle and was aware of how crucial good nutrition is in controlling Stage 3 CKD. I provided her with carefully prepared meals that were designed to fuel her body, promote her kidney health, and inspire optimism in her.

Although Cynthia's path wasn't without its challenges, with time, effort, and proper nutrition, her health started to get better. She rediscovered her zest for life as her kidney function stabilized. Her narrative serves as both a testimonial to the effectiveness of diet and nutrition in managing Stage 3 renal disease and a tale of victory over challenges.

It is key to know that Cynthia's case is not unique. Millions of people around the globe struggle with kidney disease, each with their own unique journey. This book was written for them and you.

Inside the pages of this book, you will find a wealth of information; from grasping the complexities of stage 3 kidney disease to learning the secrets of crafting a kidney-friendly diet. You will delve into the plethora of recipes created to excite your palate and care for your kidneys. You will learn the value of exercise and stress management, both of which are important pillars of kidney health.

As you travel on this journey, remember that Cynthia's case is the motivation, not the exception. It is the source of motivation for the recipes that have been painstakingly created, the inspiration for these words, and the unshakeable conviction that, armed with the appropriate information and resources, anybody can take control of their kidney health. This book is your guide, your companion, and your source of hope whether you are dealing with the challenges of chronic kidney disease or are trying to prevent it.

Welcome to a world where you have the ability to completely change the state of your kidney health. Welcome to the Recipe Cookbook for Stage 3 CKD, a comprehensive manual that encompasses nutritional guidance, meal planning, stress management tips, as well as exercise regimes to give you all the necessary tools you need to start along the path to healthier kidneys and a better future.

Let's get started!

Cheers!

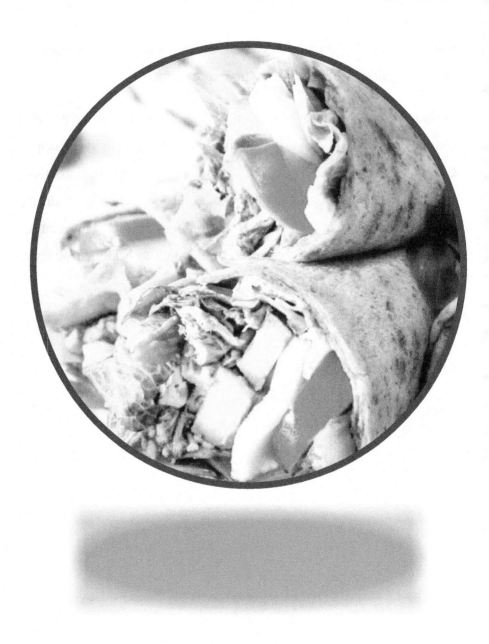

CHAPTER ONE

UNDERSTANDING STAGE 3 CHRONIC KIDNEY DISEASE

Chronic kidney disease (CKD) is a silent and progressive condition that affects the ability of the kidney to effectively filter blood. Further damage to the kidney can be prevented based on the stage of the CKD. It is categorized into stages 1 to stage 5. The former represents optimal kidney function while stage 5 shows kidney failure.

Stage 3 falls in the middle of the range. Thus, it represents a critical stage in the progression of CKD. At this stage, it's safe to say that the kidneys only have mild damage.

The function of the kidneys is measured in terms of the readings of the estimated glomerular filtration rate (eGFR), which shows how healthy or damaged a kidney is. An optimal functional kidney will have an eGFR value of more than 90, while a value less than 15 indicates stage 5 CKD. So this means the higher your eGFR, the more optimal your kidney is.

The eGFR for Stage 3 is further divided into two: 3a and 3b. The eGFR reading for 3a is between 45 - 59 eGFR, while for 3b it ranges between 30 and 44. This value suggests or shows that there is a minimal reduction in kidney function. This means while the kidney continues in its filtration of blood, this comes at a much-reduced capacity.

The core aim with stage 3 is to avert further the loss of kidney function. Clinically, this equates to averting a fall of the eGFR to the range of 29 to 15, which represents stage 4 kidney disease.

Causes and Risk Factors of Stage 3 CKD

It is crucial to comprehend the particular causes and risk factors for Stage 3 CKD. Stage 3 CKD can result from a number of reasons, including:

- **Hypertension (High Blood Pressure):** Chronically high blood pressure can harm the kidneys' tiny blood capillaries, impairing kidney function.

- **Diabetes:** Uncontrolled diabetes over time can harm the kidneys and increase the risk of developing CKD.

- **Glomerulonephritis:** Glomeruli, the kidneys' microscopic filtration units, can become inflamed and cause CKD.

- **Polycystic Kidney Disease:** A hereditary disorder that causes the kidneys to develop cysts that can affect how well they work.

Risk Factors

While some conditions can directly result in CKD, a number of risk factors increase a person's chance of getting it:

- Family History: If kidney disease runs in your family, you may be more susceptible.

- Age: People over 60 are more likely to have CKD.

- Obesity: Carrying too much body weight puts stress on the kidneys and raises the chance of developing CKD.

- Smoking: Smoking harms blood vessels throughout the body, including the kidneys.

Symptoms and Diagnosis

Symptoms

It's crucial to remember that CKD symptoms in its early stages might be subtle or even nonexistent. As kidney function deteriorates, common symptoms that may become more obvious include:

1. Fatigue: As kidney function deteriorates, the body's capacity to manufacture the hormone erythropoietin, which is in charge of producing red blood cells, is jeopardized. This may result in anemia, which causes ongoing weariness.

2. Modifications in Urination: CKD can alter the concentration of urine, which can result in abnormalities in urine volume, frequency, and color. Urine that is foamy or black may indicate renal disease.

3. Edema (swelling): Edema, especially in the ankles, legs, and hands, is caused by the retention of fluid and sodium. Also possible is facial puffiness.

4. High Blood Pressure: CKD is a cause of high blood pressure as well as a result of it. It can worsen pre-existing hypertension or, in the other direction, be made worse by it.

5. Appetite Changes: A loss of appetite and a metallic taste in the mouth are typical CKD symptoms. Also possible are nausea and vomiting.

Diagnosis

A set of tests is used to determine Stage 3 CKD diagnosis in order to assess kidney function and spot any potential complications:

eGFR: The estimated glomerular filtration rate, or eGFR, is a blood test that gauges how efficiently your kidneys are removing waste. Using your kidney function as a basis, it establishes the CKD stage.

Urinalysis: A urine test can find anomalies like blood or protein in the urine, which could mean your kidneys are damaged.

Blood pressure: Kidney problems may be indicated if blood pressure is consistently high.

Imaging Test: These may involve CT or ultrasound scans to view the kidneys and spot any structural irregularities.

The Value of Timely Intervention

Early management of Stage 3 Chronic Kidney Disease (CKD) has a major impact on the course of the condition and your quality of life. Several factors make this crucial, including:

1. **Delay the Advancement of Disease:** A critical opportunity to stop the progression of Stage 3 CKD is early detection. In order to maintain kidney function, early identification enables you to make crucial dietary and lifestyle modifications.

2. **Advanced Stages Delay:** A prompt intervention can partially reverse or stabilize Stage 3 CKD. Delaying therapy could result in more serious phases that call for more invasive procedures like dialysis or transplantation.

3. **Improving Quality of Life:** Preserving kidney function and enhancing general health are both benefits of early intervention. It takes care of complications, treats symptoms, and encourages leading a happy, active life.

4. **Lessening complications:** Cardiovascular disease and anemia are two complications that can develop from untreated CKD. Early action helps to reduce these dangers and protects your health.

5. **Personalized Treatment:** Early detection enables medical professionals to design individualized treatment regimens that are suited to your particular needs, increasing the efficacy of treatment.

6. **Enabling Self-Management:** Early intervention gives you the information and resources you need to actively control your kidney health. You may take charge of your health by learning to modify your food, way of living, and self-monitoring practices.

The Function of Diet in Stage 3 CKD Management

In managing Stage 3 Chronic Kidney Disease (CKD), diet plays a crucial and important role. Your diet has a significant and immediate impact on your general health as well as the function of your kidneys.

Appreciating the role that diet plays in controlling Stage 3 CKD requires knowledge of how diet affects renal function. Filtering waste materials and excess fluid from your blood is a crucial work done by your kidneys. Certain dietary elements, however, can either assist or overwhelm the kidneys as their function falls.

- **Sodium (Salt):** Consuming excessive amounts of sodium can cause fluid retention and elevated blood pressure, both of which can put a strain on the kidneys. Limiting salt is a goal of a kidney-friendly diet.

- **Potassium:** People with impaired renal function may have negative effects from having high blood potassium levels. To avoid harmful levels in the bloodstream, controlling potassium intake is essential.

- **Phosphorus:** Elevated phosphorus levels in CKD can be a factor in bone and cardiovascular issues. Dietary management of phosphorus intake is critical.

- **Protein:** While protein is essential for overall health, consuming too much of it can put an extra burden on the kidneys. It is frequently advised to moderate protein intake in Stage 3 CKD to alleviate this burden.

- **Fluid Balance:** While fluid is key in maintaining a healthy kidney, it is worth noting that too much of what your kidney requires can be a problem. As a result, you should monitor your fluid consumption to keep a healthy balance. This can entail modifying your fluid intake in accordance with your urine output and particular recommendations from your healthcare provider.

CHAPTER TWO

NUTRITIONAL ESSENTIALS AND MEAL PLANNING FOR STAGE 3 CKD

Key Nutrients for Kidney Health

Understanding the relevance of the following essential nutrients is crucial before starting your journey to better kidney health:

Protein: Protein is important for overall health, but in Stage 3 CKD, moderation is key. The normal range for the daily recommended protein intake is 0.6 to 0.8 grams of protein per kilogram of body weight. Lean meats (such as chicken and turkey), fish, eggs, and plant-based choices like tofu and lentils are all excellent sources of protein. Your precise protein objectives should decide the portion sizes you consume.

Sodium (Salt): To maintain healthy kidneys, sodium intake must be kept to a minimum. Depending on individual needs, the recommended daily salt intake ranges from 1,500 to 2,300 milligrams. Concentrate on eating fresh, healthy foods and add herbs and spices for flavor to limit sodium intake. Avoid restaurant dishes and processed foods with high sodium.

Potassium: It's important to control potassium levels, and 2,000 to 3,000 milligrams per day is usually the recommended amount. Bananas, potatoes, and oranges are high-potassium foods that should be avoided. Potassium concentration can be decreased through cooking processes including leaching (soaking in water).

Phosphorus: Daily phosphorus requirements typically range from 800 to 1,000 milligrams, and intake should be regularly monitored. Limit your intake of high-phosphorus foods like dairy, almonds, and some meats. Understanding the phosphorus content of foods requires reading the food labels. Phosphate binders may be suggested by your dietician to successfully manage phosphorus levels.

Managing Sodium, Potassium, and Phosphorus Intake

Maintaining kidney health requires careful monitoring of salt, potassium, and phosphorus consumption. Here is a list of helpful tips for each of these vital nutrients, broken down succinctly:

Controlling Sodium

For healthy kidney function, salt intake must be reduced. You may rely on home-cooked meals and fresh ingredients to succeed in this. Take advantage of the naturally low-sodium fresh vegetables, lean meats, and entire grains. Dump the salt at home and experiment with herbs and spices to flavor your food in unique ways. Because you have control over the products and flavors when you cook at home, you can reduce your sodium intake. When eating out, exercise caution because many restaurant foods include a lot of sodium.

Choose restaurants that use low-sodium alternatives or ask about the salt content.

Management of Potassium:

It's important to balance your potassium intake, especially if you have impaired kidney function. Identify foods high in potassium, such as bananas, oranges, potatoes, and tomatoes. While healthy, moderation is essential. Watch your portion amounts, especially when eating foods high in potassium. Learn about cooking methods that lower potassium in vegetables, such as leaching. Create a customized potassium management strategy that is based on your tastes and your dietary requirements.

Phosphorus Management

Controlling phosphorus intake is crucial since increased phosphorus levels can exacerbate CKD problems. Make it a practice to study food labels to determine the amount of phosphorus in packaged foods, paying close attention to words like "phosphate" or "phosphoric acid." Reduce your intake of processed foods, which frequently have additives containing phosphorus.

Tips For Designing a Stage 3 CKD Meal Plan

Creating a diet plan for those with Stage 3 CKD is a critical first step toward improving renal function. Your meal plan should be customized to meet your unique dietary demands and restrictions with an emphasis on maintaining renal function. The following tips will help you create a diet that is appropriate for maintaining kidney health:

1. Maintaining Balance: A balanced diet should be part of a well-rounded meal plan. Aim to include all necessary nutrients while adhering to guidelines for protein, salt, potassium, and phosphorus. This balance helps to support your kidneys and upholds your overall health.

2. Meal Frequency and Time: Take into account the frequency and time of your meals. Getting enough nutrients throughout the day can improve kidney function and help control blood sugar levels. Your healthcare professional can give you advice on the frequency and portion you require.

3. Dietary Restrictions: Choose kidney-friendly meals that fit your dietary needs. Fish, chicken, turkey, and plant-based substitutes are all excellent sources of lean protein. Choose whole grains, and emphasize fruit and non-starchy vegetables. Reduce your intake of foods heavy in potassium, phosphorus, and sodium.

4. Mindful Cooking Method: Cooking methods that use less salt or fat, such as grilling, broiling, and baking, are preferable to frying. Vegetables high in potassium may be lessened by leaching.

5. Portion Control: Managing nutritional intake requires good portion management. Learn how to divide your plate into portions for vegetables, lean protein, and carbohydrates using the "plate method." Most often, it is advised to weigh and measure food to achieve precise portion control.

6. Snacking Wisely: If you plan to snack between meals, select kidney-friendly options. Yogurt, fresh fruit, unsalted nuts, and low-phosphorus crackers are good alternatives. Be sure to portion these snacks wisely to meet your dietary objectives.

7. Keep a Record: To keep track of your daily nutritional consumption, think about maintaining a food journal. This might be a useful tool for you to track your development and make the necessary changes to your food plan.

Smart Shopping Tips

It may first seem difficult to shop at the grocery store with a focus on kidney-friendly items, but with the appropriate techniques, you can confidently stock your basket with foods that support your Stage 3 CKD meal plan. Here is a thorough examination of how to choose kidney-friendly items when supermarket shopping:

1. **Plan ahead:** Before you go shopping, ensure you plan your meals for the subsequent weeks. Depending on your menu plan, let your shopping list capture all the needed ingredients. The advantage this has is that it helps you to be organized and also avoids the temptation of impulsive purchases.

2. **Read Food Labels:** When it comes to shopping for kidney-friendly items, food labels are your greatest friend. Pay particular attention to products with the designations "low sodium" or "no salt added." You can find phosphorus additions in packaged foods such as "phosphate" or "phosphoric acid" in the ingredients list. Understanding these concepts will help you make wise decisions.

3. **Go Fresh and Frozen:** Choose fresh fruits and vegetables, lean meats, and canned or frozen items that are low-sodium. The sodium content of fresh produce is frequently lower than that of canned food. Pick lean beef and chicken cuts, and think about seafood options high in omega-3 fatty acids, including salmon or trout.

4. **Limit Processed Foods:** Convenience and highly processed foods may contain salt and phosphorus that are hidden in the ingredients. Reduce how often you consume these foods since they can easily cause you to eat more than is allowed for you. Choose whole, unprocessed foods as a substitute.

5. **Avoid Excessive Seasonings:** Fresh herbs and spices are a great way to flavor food without adding sodium, but be careful when using seasoning blends since some may have excessive salt content. Ensure to read the labels on these spices and choose the low-sodium options.

6. **Make Bulk Purchases:** Whole grains and legumes are two examples of staple foods that can be economical and practical to buy in bulk. To prevent overconsumption, make sure your storage is big enough and think about portioning out bulk items.

Meal Prep Strategies for Convenience

Effective meal prep is key in the quest to maintain a healthy kidney diet. Strategizing out ways to make meals ahead of time will ensure your journey is simplified and you readily have kidney-friendly options at your disposal. Here are some strategies to help you achieve this with ease.

1. **Batch Cooking:** You can save yourself time and effort if you make large amounts of kidney-friendly diets. After the meal preparation, divide it into servings, and put them in the freezer for later use. Apart from saving you the stress of cooking daily, it also ensures you readily have healthy meals at your convenience.

2. **Pre-cut and Pre-packaged:** Simplify the process of preparing your meals by pre-cutting vegetables and measuring out snacks in advance. With these items being readily at your disposal, it makes it easier for you to include them in your meals. More than that, it also guarantees that you are consuming freshly made kidney ingredients.

3. **Invest in Kitchen Gadgets:** Slow cookers or pressure cookers are invaluable investments for your kitchen. Investing in these gadgets goes a long way to simplify your meal preparation process. These appliances serve you time and also make your cooking efforts minimal, thus making for efficient meal prep.

4. **Label and Date:** Ensure to label and date your meals after batch cooking and freezing. This makes it easier for you to readily identify any item and track same for freshness. To preserve the quality of your meals, use freezer-safe containers or bags.

5. **Portion Control:** Practice dividing your meals into suitable serving sizes. This makes it easy for you to reach out for a meal at your convenience; it also helps you to manage portion control. Tracking your intake of sodium, potassium, and phosphorus levels is made easier with portioning.

6. **Create Weekly Plans:** Make weekly menu plans that capture a range of kidney-friendly recipes. A menu in place streamlines grocery shopping and dictates meal preparation, resulting in a completely healthy diet.

7. **Maintain a Well-Stocked Pantry:** Keep your pantry stocked with essential ingredients like whole grains, low-salt broths, and canned vegetables with no added sodium. This makes sure you have the core ingredients available for your meal prep.

CHAPTER THREE

BREAKFAST RECIPES

Vegetable Omelette

Prep Time: 10 minutes Cook Time: 10 minutes Servings: 2

Ingredients:

- 4 large eggs
- 1/4 cup chopped bell peppers
- 1/4 cup diced tomatoes
- 1/4 cup chopped onions
- 2 tbsp sliced fresh herbs (such as chives or parsley)
- 1 tbsp olive oil
- 2 tbsps low-fat cheese
- Salt and pepper to taste

Directions:

1. In a basin, beat the eggs and season same with pepper and salt.
2. Over medium heat in a non-stick skillet, heat the olive oil. Then put in the onions, chopped peppers, and tomatoes. Fry until it softens.
3. Decant the beaten eggs atop the vegetables and cook until set.
4. Scatter the cheese and fresh herbs atop the mixture.
5. Fold the omelette in half, and serve.

Nutritional Information (per serving):

Calories: 180 Protein: 13g Sodium: 220mg Fiber: 2g Potassium: 250mg Phosphorus: 150mg Carbs: 4g

Greek Yogurt Parfait

Prep Time: 5 minutes Servings: 1

Ingredients:
- 1/2 cup plain Greek yogurt
- 1/4 cup fresh berries (example: strawberries or blueberries)
- 1 tbsp chopped almonds
- 1 tbsp honey (optional)

Directions:
1. Get ready a glass and pour in the low-fat Greek yogurt.
2. Atop the yoghurt, layer the assorted berries.
3. Evenly scatter the diced almonds atop the berries.
4. For more sweetness, you can sprinkle honey over it
5. Go over the same process for the leftover ingredients, making a visually attractive parfait.
6. Serve immediately and enjoy!

Nutritional Information (per serving):
Calories: 220 Protein: 18g Sodium: 60mg Fiber: 3g Potassium: 260mg Phosphorus: 170mg Carbs: 18g

Spinach and Feta Scramble

Prep Time: 10 minutes Cook Time: 10 minutes Servings: 2

Ingredients:
- 4 large eggs
- 1 cup fresh spinach leaves
- 1/4 cup crumbled feta cheese
- 1 tbsp olive oil
- Salt and pepper to taste

Directions:
1. Over medium heat in a non-stick skillet, heat the olive oil. Then put in the spinach and have it sautéed until it wilts.
2. In a small, beat the eggs and spice up with pepper and salt.

3. Decant the beaten eggs into the spinach mixture in the skillet. Cook for approximately 2-3 minutes
4. Include the crumbled feta cheese and scramble until they are done to your satisfaction.

Nutritional Information (per serving):

Calories: 260 Protein: 17g Sodium: 360mg Fiber: 1g Potassium: 230mg Phosphorus: 270mg Carbs: 2g

Banana Nut Oatmeal

Prep Time: 5 minutes Cook Time: 10 minutes Servings: 2

Ingredients:

- 1 cup oats
- 2 cups water
- 1 ripe banana, mashed
- 1/4 cup chopped walnuts
- 1 tbsp cinnamon
- 1 tbsp honey (optional)

Directions:

1. Put water in a saucepan and bring to a boil. Add and stir the oats and lower the heat to a simmer.
2. Stirring regularly, cook for 5-7 minutes or until the oats are cooked and most of the liquid has been absorbed.
3. Turn off the heat and add the cinnamon, mashed banana, and sliced walnuts.
4. If you desire, sprinkle honey atop it.

Nutritional Information (per serving):

Calories: 280 Protein: 7g Sodium: 5mg Fiber: 6g Potassium: 280mg Phosphorus: 120mg Carbs: 50g

Spinach and Tomato Breakfast Quesadilla

Prep Time: 10 minutes Cook Time: 10 minutes Servings: 2

Ingredients:

- 2 whole wheat tortillas
- 4 large eggs, beaten
- 1 cup fresh spinach leaves
- 1/2 cup diced tomatoes
- Cooking spray
- 1/4 cup shredded low-sodium mozzarella cheese
- Salt and pepper to taste

Directions:

1. In a basin, beat the eggs and season same with pepper and salt.
2. Over medium heat in a non-stick skillet, cook the whisked eggs until they start to set.
3. Pour the chopped tomatoes and spinach into the egg mixture. Cook this till the eggs are fully cooked.
4. Place half of the egg mixture atop one of the tortillas in the skillet, then top with half of the mozzarella cheese. Finally, top with the second tortilla.
5. Cook, flipping halfway through, until the tortillas are brown and the cheese is melted.
6. Do the same for the second quesadilla. Slice and serve.

Nutritional Information (per serving):

Calories: 320 Protein: 17g Sodium: 410mg Fiber: 3g Potassium: 240mg Phosphorus: 220mg Carbs: 27g

Berry Protein Smoothie

Prep Time: 5 minutes Servings: 1

Ingredients:

- 1/2 cup low-fat yogurt
- 1/2 cup unsweetened almond milk
- 1/2 cup assorted berries (e.g., blueberries, raspberries)
- 1 spoon of low-phosphorus protein powder
- 1 tbsp chia seeds (optional)

Directions:

1. Combine yogurt, almond milk, mixed berries, protein powder, and chia seeds in a blender.
2. Blend until smooth and creamy.

Nutritional Information (per serving):

Calories: 250 Protein: 25g Sodium: 180mg Fiber: 6g Potassium: 230mg Phosphorus: 160mg Carbs: 30g

Avocado Toast with Poached Egg

Prep Time: 10 minutes Cook Time: 5 minutes Servings: 2

Ingredients:

- 2 slices whole wheat bread, toasted
- 1 ripe avocado
- 2 large eggs, poached
- 1/2 tbsp white vinegar (for poaching)
- Salt and pepper to taste
- Fresh herbs (parsley or chives) for garnish (optional)

Directions:

1. Toast the whole-wheat bread until it reaches the required crispness.
2. Split the avocado in half, mash one-half, and season with salt and pepper.

3. Bring water to a medium simmer in a saucepan and add the white vinegar. Then, break the eggs into a small dish and gently pour same into the boiling water, and let it cook for approximately 2-3 minutes to form a firm yolk.
4. Top the avocado-topped bread with poached eggs.
5. Add pepper and salt to taste.
6. As desired, use parsley or chives for garnishing.
7. Serve immediately.

Nutritional Information (per serving):

Calories: 280 Protein: 13g Sodium: 160mg Fiber: 7g Potassium: 480mg Phosphorus: 200mg Carbs: 19g

Spinach and Mushroom Breakfast Wrap

Prep Time: 10 minutes Cook Time: 10 minutes Servings: 2

Ingredients:
- 2 whole wheat tortillas
- 4 large eggs, beaten
- 1 cup fresh spinach leaves
- 1/2 cup sliced mushrooms
- 1/4 cup diced onions
- 1/4 cup shredded low-sodium cheddar cheese
- Salt and pepper to taste
- Cooking Spray

Directions:
1. In a small dish, beat the eggs and season with salt and pepper
2. Over a medium heat, heat the non-stick skillet and lightly coat with the cooking spray
3. Add spinach, sliced mushrooms, and diced onions to the skillet. Continue cooking until they are tender.
4. Pour in the whisked eggs and cook till the eggs start to set.

5. Place one tortilla in the skillet, add half of the egg mixture on top, sprinkle with half of the cheddar cheese, and cover with the second tortilla.
6. Cook until tortillas are golden and cheese is melted, flipping halfway through.
7. Repeat for the second wrap. Slice and serve.

Nutritional Information (per serving):
Calories: 330 Protein: 19g Sodium: 320mg Fiber: 6g Potassium: 340mg Phosphorus: 240mg Carbs: 21g

Cottage Cheese Pancakes

Prep Time: 10 minutes Cook Time: 10 minutes Servings: 2

Ingredients:
- 1 cup low-fat cottage cheese
- 2 large eggs
- 1/4 cup whole wheat flour
- 1/4 tbsp baking powder
- 1/2 tbsp vanilla extract
- Cooking Spray
- 1/2 cup fresh berries (e.g., raspberries or blueberries)

Directions:
1. In a basin, thoroughly mix together the whole wheat flour, cottage cheese, eggs, vanilla extract, and baking powder.
2. Over a medium heat, heat a non-stick skillet and use the cooking spray to lightly grease it.
3. For each pancake, add 1/4 cup of the pancake batter to the skillet. Cook until surface bubbles appear, then flip and continue cooking until both sides are brown.
4. Carry out step 4 with the remaining batter.
5. Serve with fresh berries.

Nutritional Information (per serving):

Calories: 260 Protein: 24g Sodium: 440mg Fiber: 3g Potassium: 300mg Phosphorus: 260mg Carbs: 20g

Peanut Butter Banana Smoothie Bowl

Prep Time: 10 minutes Servings: 1

Ingredients:

- 1 ripe banana
- 2 tbsps peanut butter
- 1/2 cup unsweetened almond milk
- 1/4 cup low-fat Greek yogurt
- 1 tbsp chia seeds
- Sliced banana and chopped nuts for topping

Directions:

1. In a blender, add the Greek yogurt, ripe banana, peanut butter, chia seeds, and almond milk.
2. Blend until smooth and creamy.
3. Pour the smoothie into a bowl, then top with chopped nuts and banana slices.

Nutritional Information (per serving):

Calories: 390 Protein: 15g Sodium: 170mg Fiber: 9g Potassium: 570mg Phosphorus: 250mg Carbs: 40g

CHAPTER FOUR

LUNCH RECIPES

Grilled Chicken and Vegetable Salad

Prep Time: 15 minutes Cook Time: 15 minutes Servings: 2

Ingredients:
- 2 chicken breasts (boneless and skinless)
- 4 cups assorted salad greens
- 1 cup cherry tomatoes, halved
- 1/2 cucumber, sliced
- 1/4 cup red onion, thinly sliced
- 2 tbsps balsamic vinaigrette dressing (low-sodium)
- Salt and pepper to taste

Directions:
1. Use pepper and salt to season the chicken breasts, then grill until cooked through.
2. Make thin strips from the grilled chicken.
3. In a large basin, mix together the cherry tomatoes, red onion, cucumber, and salad greens.
4. Place the chicken strips atop the salad mixture and then sprinkle with balsamic vinaigrette dressing.
5. Toss gently to combine.

Nutritional Information (per serving):
Calories: 320 Protein: 30g Sodium: 180mg Fiber: 4g Potassium: 650mg Phosphorus: 280mg Carbs: 12g

Quinoa and Black Bean Salad

Prep Time: 15 minutes Cook Time: 15 minutes Servings: 4

Ingredients:

- 1 cup quinoa, rinsed
- 2 cups low-sodium vegetable broth
- Drained and rinsed black beans (1 can -n15 oz),
- fresh or frozen corn kernels (1 cup)
- 1/2 cup chopped bell peppers (whichever color)
- 1/4 cup sliced cilantro
- 2 tbsps olive oil
- Juice of 1 lime
- Salt and pepper to taste

Directions:

1. In a saucepan, bring vegetable broth to a boil, then put the quinoa. Lower heat, cover, and cook for about 15 minutes or until quinoa is cooked and liquid is absorbed.
2. In a large dish, mix together the cooked quinoa, cilantro, corn, black beans, and bell peppers.
3. In a small basin, meld together the lime juice, pepper, olive oil, and salt.
4. Sprinkle over the salad and lob to coat.

Nutritional Information (per serving):

Calories: 300 Protein: 9g Sodium: 200mg Fiber: 6g Potassium: 280mg Phosphorus: 150mg Carbs: 52g

Tuna and White Bean Salad

Prep Time: 10 minutes Servings: 2

Ingredients:

- 1 can (5 oz) low-sodium tuna, drained
- 1 can (15 oz) white beans (cannellini or navy), drained and rinsed

- 1/4 cup chopped red onion
- 1/4 cup diced parsley
- 2 tbsps olive oil
- 1 tbsp lemon juice
- Salt and pepper to taste

Directions:
1. In a big basin, mix together white beans, drained tuna, chopped parsley, and red onion.
2. In a small basin, meld together lemon juice, pepper, olive oil, and salt. Drizzle over the salad and lob to combine.

Nutritional Information (per serving):
Calories: 340 Protein: 22g Sodium: 170mg Fiber: 10g Potassium: 530mg Phosphorus: 260mg Carbs: 38g

Spinach and Mushroom Stuffed Chicken Breast

Prep Time: 20 minutes Cook Time: 25 minutes Servings: 2

Ingredients:
- 2 chicken breasts (boneless and skinless)
- 1 cup fresh spinach leaves
- 1/2 cup chopped mushrooms
- 1/4 cup low-sodium chicken broth
- 2 tbsps grated Parmesan cheese
- 1 tbsp olive oil
- Salt and pepper to taste

Directions:
1. Preheat the oven to a Fahrenheit degree of 375.
2. Over a medium heat in a skillet, heat the olive oil. Put in the chopped mushrooms and sauté until they release their moisture.
3. Put fresh spinach and chicken broth in the skillet. Cook until the broth is reduced and the spinach wilts.

4. Slice a pocket into each chicken breast and fill it with the spinach and mushroom blend.
5. Season chicken breasts with salt and pepper, then place in a baking tray.
6. Top the chicken with grated Parmesan cheese.
7. Bake for 25 minutes or until the chicken is cooked through.

Nutritional Information (per serving):

Calories: 280 Protein: 40g Sodium: 220mg Fiber: 2g Potassium: 640mg Phosphorus: 310mg Carbs: 4g

Lentil and Vegetable Soup

Prep Time: 10 minutes Cook Time: 30 minutes Servings: 4

Ingredients:

- Rinsed, dried brown or green lentils (1 cup)
- 4 cups low-sodium vegetable broth
- 1 cup diced carrots
- 1 cup diced celery
- 1 cup diced onion
- 2 cloves garlic, minced
- 1 tbsp olive oil
- 1 bay leaf
- 1 tbsp dried thyme
- Salt and pepper to taste

Directions:

1. Over a medium heat in a large pot, heat the olive oil. Include diced onion, celery, carrots, and garlic. Sauté until vegetables begin to soften.
2. Add rinsed lentils, vegetable broth, bay leaf, dried thyme, salt, and pepper to the pot.
3. Bring the mixture to a boil before lowering the heat to a simmer. Cover and allow it to cook for about 30 minutes or until lentils turn tender.

4. Remove the bay leaf before serving.

Nutritional Information (per serving):

Calories: 280 Protein: 18g Sodium: 400mg Fiber: 14g Potassium: 570mg Phosphorus: 360mg Carbs: 46g

Turkey and Avocado Wrap

Prep Time: 10 minutes Servings: 2

Ingredients:

- 4 oz low-sodium turkey breast slices
- 1 ripe avocado, sliced
- 2 whole wheat tortillas
- 1/2 cup mixed greens
- 2 tbsps low-fat Greek yogurt
- 1 tbsp Dijon mustard

Directions:

1. Combine Greek yogurt and Dijon mustard in a small bowl.
2. Spread the yogurt-mustard mixture over each of the whole-wheat tortillas.
3. Layer mixed greens, turkey slices, and avocado slices on the tortillas.
4. Roll up the tortillas into wraps and serve.

Nutritional Information (per serving):

Calories: 330 Protein: 18g Sodium: 210mg Fiber: 9g Potassium: 510mg Phosphorus: 230mg Carbs: 31g

Vegetable Stir-Fry

Prep Time: 15 minutes Cook Time: 15 minutes Servings: 4

Ingredients:

- 2 cups assorted vegetables (such as snap peas, broccoli, bell peppers)
- 1 cup sliced mushrooms

- 1 cup sliced carrots
- 1/2 cup sliced red onion
- 2 cloves garlic, minced
- 2 tbsps low-sodium stir-fry sauce
- 1 tbsp olive oil
- 1 cup cooked brown rice

Directions:

1. In a sizable skillet or wok, heat the olive oil over high heat.
2. Include red onion slices and minced garlic. Stir-fry for about 1-2 minutes.
3. Include carrots, mushrooms, and mixed veggies. Stir-fry for 5-7 minutes until veggies are crisp-tender.
4. Add the low-sodium stir-fry sauce and simmer for an additional two minutes.
5. Serve the stir-fry over cooked brown rice.

Nutritional Information (per serving):

Calories: 290 Protein: 7g Sodium: 160mg Fiber: 5g Potassium: 460mg Phosphorus: 120mg Carbs: 52g

Baked Salmon with Lemon-Dill Sauce

Prep Time: 10 minutes Cook Time: 20 minutes Servings: 2

Ingredients:

- 2 salmon fillets (6 oz each)
- 1 lemon, sliced
- 2 tbsps fresh dill, chopped
- 2 tbsps low-fat mayonnaise
- 1 tbsp Dijon mustard
- Salt and pepper to taste

Directions:

1. Preheat the oven to a Fahrenheit temperature of 375°F
2. Arrange the salmon fillets on a baking pan covered with foil.
3. Arrange the salmon fillets on a foiled-lined baking sheet.

4. Spice the salmon with salt and pepper, then top with lemon slices and half of the diced dill.
5. Bake the salmon for 15-20 minutes, or until it flakes with a fork with ease.
6. In a small basin, mix low-fat mayonnaise, Dijon mustard, and the left over chopped dill.
7. Serve the baked salmon with lemon-dill sauce.

Nutritional Information (per serving):
Calories: 320 Protein: 36g Sodium: 210mg Fiber: 2g Potassium: 760mg Phosphorus: 360mg Carbs: 5g

Eggplant and Tomato Stew

Prep Time: 15 minutes Cook Time: 30 minutes Servings: 4

Ingredients:
- 1 large eggplant, diced
- Low-salt chopped tomatoes (1 can -15 oz)
- 1 cup diced bell peppers (any color)
- 1 cup diced onions
- 2 cloves garlic, minced
- 2 tbsps olive oil
- 1 tbsp dried basil
- Salt and pepper to taste

Directions:
1. Over a medium heat, heat the olive oil in a large pot. Add diced onions and garlic. Sauté until onions become translucent.
2. Add chopped eggplant, dried basil, bell peppers, chopped tomatoes, pepper and salt to the pot. Stir to combine.
3. Cover and simmer for 30 minutes or until eggplant is tender.
4. Serve hot.

Nutritional Information (per serving):

Calories: 200 Protein: 3g Sodium: 220mg Fiber: 7g Potassium: 680mg Phosphorus: 80mg Carbs: 31g

Veggie and Hummus Wrap

Prep Time: 10 minutes Servings: 2

Ingredients:

- 2 whole wheat tortillas
- 1/2 cup hummus
- 1 cup mixed salad greens
- 1/2 cup sliced cucumber
- 1/2 cup cut bell peppers (whichever color)
- 1/4 cup shredded carrots

Directions:

1. Arrange whole wheat tortillas and evenly spread each with hummus.
2. Spread salad greens, cukes, bell peppers, and carrots on the tortillas.
3. Create wraps out of the tortillas and serve.

Nutritional Information (per serving):

Calories: 260 Protein: 7g Sodium: 410mg Fiber: 8g Potassium: 360mg Phosphorus: 180mg Carbs: 36g

CHAPTER FIVE

DINNER RECIPES

Lemon Herb Grilled Chicken

Prep Time: 10 minutes Cook Time: 15 minutes Servings: 2

Ingredients:
- 2 chicken breasts (boneless and skinless)
- 1 lemon, juiced and zested
- 2 cloves garlic, minced
- 1 tbsp fresh parsley, minced
- 1 tbsp fresh thyme, minced
- 1 tbsp olive oil
- Salt and pepper to taste

Directions:
1. In a basin, mix together the minced garlic, chopped thyme, lemon juice, olive oil, chopped parsley, lemon zest, salt, and pepper.
2. Put the chicken breasts in a ziplock bag and decant the marinade upon them. Seal the bag and put it in the refrigerator for not less than 30 minutes.
3. Set the grill to medium-high heat. Grill chicken for 6 to 8 minutes on each side, or until well done.
4. Serve hot.

Nutritional Information (per serving):
Calories: 220 Protein: 40g Sodium: 95mg Fiber: 1g Potassium: 350mg Phosphorus: 250mg Carbs: 3g

Baked Cod with Tomato-Basil Sauce

Prep Time: 15 minutes Cook Time: 20 minutes Servings: 2

Ingredients:
- 2 cod fillets (6 oz each)
- 1 cup chopped tomatoes (canned, unsalted)
- 1/4 cup fresh basil, chopped
- 2 cloves garlic, diced
- 1 tbsp olive oil
- Salt and pepper to taste

Directions:
1. Preheat the oven to a Fahrenheit degree of 375°F.
2. Over a medium heat, heat the olive oil in a skillet. Pour in diced garlic and sauté for approximately 1 minute.
3. Include the chopped tomatoes and diced basil in the skillet. Cook for an extra 3-5 minutes until well heated.
4. Use pepper and salt to season the cod fillets, then set them in a baking bowl.
5. Pour the tomato-basil sauce over the cod.
6. Cook for about 15-20 minutes or until the cod flakes with a fork without difficulty.
7. Serve with sauce.

Nutritional Information (per serving):
Calories: 250 Protein: 38g Sodium: 180mg Fiber: 2g Potassium: 680mg Phosphorus: 330mg Carbs: 5g

Vegetable and Chickpea Stir-Fry

Prep Time: 15 minutes Cook Time: 15 minutes Servings: 4

Ingredients:
- 2 cups diverse vegetables (such as snap peas, broccoli, bell peppers)
- 1 can (15 oz) low-sodium chickpeas, drained and rinsed

- 1 cup cut mushrooms
- 1/2 cup divided red onion
- 2 cloves garlic, shredded
- 2 tbsps low-sodium stir-fry sauce
- 1 tbsp olive oil
- 2 cups cooked brown rice

Directions:

1. In a sizable skillet or wok, heat the olive oil over high heat.
2. Include red onion slices and minced garlic. Stir-fry for about 1 -2 minutes.
3. Include chickpeas, sliced mushrooms, and assorted vegetables. Stir-fry for 5-7 minutes or until the veggies are crisp-tender.
4. Add the low-sodium stir-fry sauce, then simmer for an additional two minutes.
5. Serve atop cooked brown rice.

Nutritional Information (per serving):

Calories: 280 Protein: 9g Sodium: 180mg Fiber: 7g Potassium: 470mg Phosphorus: 170mg Carbs: 52g

Quinoa and Vegetable Pilaf

Prep Time: 15 minutes Cook Time: 20 minutes Servings: 4

Ingredients:

- 1 cup quinoa, rinsed
- 2 cups low-sodium vegetable broth
- 2 cups mixed vegetables (e.g., carrots, peas, corn)
- 1/4 cup chopped onions
- 2 cloves garlic, shredded
- 1 tbsp olive oil
- 1/4 cup cut fresh parsley
- Salt and pepper to taste

Directions:

1. In a saucepan over medium heat, heat the olive. Add minced garlic and diced onions. Allow the onions to be sautéed until transparent.
2. Add to the saucepan the vegetable broth and quinoa. Allow to a boil, and reduce the heat to a simmer. Cover the pan and cook same for about 15-20 minutes or until the quinoa liquid has been absorbed.
3. In a different pot, steam or boil assorted vegetables until tender.
4. Stir cooked vegetables and chopped parsley into the quinoa after fluffing it with a fork.
5. Spice it up with pepper and salt before serving.

Nutritional Information (per serving):

Calories: 260 Protein: 8g Sodium: 210mg Fiber: 5g Potassium: 400mg Phosphorus: 160mg Carbs: 45g

Turkey and Vegetable Skewers

Prep Time: 15 minutes Cook Time: 10 minutes Servings: 4

Ingredients:

- 1 lb turkey breast, divided into bits
- 2 cups mixed vegetables (e.g., bell peppers, zucchini, cherry tomatoes)
- 2 tbsps olive oil
- 1 tbsp dried oregano
- Salt and pepper to taste

Directions:

1. Turn on the grill to a medium-high setting.
2. Thread chopped turkey and vegetable varieties onto skewers.
3. Combine the olive oil, salt, pepper, and dried oregano in a small bowl.
4. Apply the olive oil to the skewers.

5. On each side, grill skewers for approximately 4-5 minutes or until the turkey is fully cooked and the vegetables turn charred.
6. Serve hot.

Nutritional Information (per serving):
Calories: 240 Protein: 30g Sodium: 70mg Fiber: 4g Potassium: 480mg Phosphorus: 250mg Carbs: 10g

Lentil and Vegetable Stir-Fry

Prep Time: 15 minutes Cook Time: 20 minutes Servings: 4

Ingredients:
- Rinsed, dried brown or green lentils(1 cup)
- 4 cups low-sodium vegetable broth
- 2 cups mixed vegetables (such as snap peas, broccoli, bell peppers,)
- 1 cup cut mushrooms
- 1/2 cup sliced red onion
- 2 cloves garlic, shredded
- 2 tbsps low-sodium stir-fry sauce
- 1 tbsp olive oil

Directions:
1. Pour the vegetable broth into the saucepan and bring to a boil. Include the lentils, then cover and lower the heat to simmer for about 20 minutes or until the lentils are tender.
2. In a sizable skillet or wok, heat the olive oil over high heat.
3. Include red onion slices and minced garlic. Stir-fry for 1-2 minutes.
4. Include low-sodium stir-fry sauce, sliced mushrooms, and mixed vegetables. Stir-fry for 5-7 minutes until vegetables turn crisp-tender.
5. Serve the stir-fry over cooked lentils.

Nutritional Information (per serving):
Calories: 290 Protein: 16g Sodium: 420mg Fiber: 12g Potassium: 620mg Phosphorus: 280mg Carbs: 51g

Spinach and Mushroom Stuffed Bell Peppers

Prep Time: 20 minutes Cook Time: 35 minutes Servings: 4

Ingredients:
- 4 bell peppers (any color)
- 2 cups fresh spinach leaves
- 1 cup cut mushrooms
- 1/2 cup chopped tomatoes (canned, no salt added)
- 1/2 cup cooked quinoa
- 1/4 cup chopped onions
- 2 cloves garlic, minced
- 1 tbsp olive oil
- 1/2 tbsp dried basil
- 1/2 tbsp dried oregano
- Salt and pepper to taste

Directions:
1. Preheat the oven to a Fahrenheit degree of 375.
2. Cut off the top of the bell peppers and take out the seeds and membranes.
3. Over a medium heat, heat olive oil in a skillet. Add chopped onions and minced garlic. Sauté until onions turn translucent.
4. Pour the cut mushrooms and chopped tomatoes into the skillet. Cook for approximately 3-5 minutes.
5. Add fresh spinach and stir until it wilts.
6. Turn off the heat and stir in cooked quinoa, along with the salt, pepper, dried basil, and dried oregano.
7. Stuff the bell peppers with the blend and put them in a baking bowl.
8. Bake the bell peppers for 30-35 minutes, or until they are tender.

Nutritional Information (per serving):
Calories: 200 Protein: 6g Sodium: 30mg Fiber: 6g Potassium: 570mg Phosphorus: 110mg Carbs: 39g

Pork Tenderloin with Roasted Vegetables

Prep Time: 15 minutes Cook Time: 30 minutes Servings: 2

Ingredients:
- 1 pork tenderloin (about 12 oz)
- 2 cups assorted vegetables (such as red potatoes, carrots, brussels sprouts)
- 1 tbsp olive oil
- 1 tbsp dried rosemary
- 1/2 tbsp dried thyme
- Salt and pepper to taste

Directions:
1. Set the oven temperature to 425°F (220°C).
2. Combine mixed vegetables in a large bowl with the olive oil, salt, pepper, dried thyme, and rosemary.
3. Center the pork tenderloin on a baking sheet and surround it with vegetables.
4. Roast in the oven for approximately 25-30 minutes or until the pork reaches a temperature of 145°F (63°C).
5. Take it out from the oven and allow it a few minutes to rest before slicing.
6. Serve with roasted vegetables.

Nutritional Information (per serving):
Calories: 300 Protein: 30g Sodium: 70mg Fiber: 6g Potassium: 670mg Phosphorus: 230mg Carbs: 20g

Turkey Meatballs with Zucchini Noodles

Prep Time: 20 minutes Cook Time: 25 minutes Servings: 4

Ingredients:

- 1 lb lean ground turkey
- 1/4 cup whole wheat breadcrumbs
- 1/4 cup grated Parmesan cheese
- 1/4 cup chopped fresh parsley
- 1 egg
- 1 clove garlic, minced
- 4 medium zucchini, spiralized into noodles
- 1 cup low-sodium marinara sauce
- 1 tbsp olive oil
- Salt and pepper to taste

Directions:

1. Combine egg, minced garlic, salt, and pepper in a bowl along with lean ground turkey, whole wheat breadcrumbs, grated Parmesan cheese, and fresh parsley. Combine thoroughly after mixing.
2. Create meatballs out of the mixture.
3. Set a large skillet over medium-high heat to warm the olive oil. Add the meatballs and cook for 10 to 15 minutes, or until thoroughly browned.
4. Spiralize zucchini to create noodles while the meatballs are cooking.
5. Bring marinara sauce to a boil in a different skillet. Add the zucchini noodles, and cook for an additional three to five minutes, or until done.
6. Serve turkey meatballs atop zucchini noodles.

Nutritional Information (per serving):

Calories: 280 Protein: 28g Sodium: 380mg Fiber: 4g Potassium: 930mg Phosphorus: 330mg Carbs: 14g

Veggie and Brown Rice Bowl

Prep Time: 15 minutes Cook Time: 20 minutes Servings: 4

Ingredients:

- 2 cups cooked brown rice
- 2 cups varied vegetables (e.g., broccoli, bell peppers, snap peas)
- 1 cup cut mushrooms
- 1/2 cup chopped onions
- 2 cloves garlic, minced
- 2 tbsps low-sodium stir-fry sauce
- 1 tbsp olive oil

Directions:

1. Over a high heat, heat the olive oil in a skillet.
2. Include minced garlic and chopped onions. Stir-fry for 1-2 minutes.
3. Include low-sodium stir-fry sauce, cut mushrooms, and assorted vegetables. Stir-fry for 5-7 minutes until vegetables become crisp-tender.
4. Serve the stir-fry over cooked brown rice.

Nutritional Information (per serving):

Calories: 260 Protein: 5g Sodium: 320mg Fiber: 4g Potassium: 380mg Phosphorus: 140mg Carbs: 53g

CHAPTER SIX

SNACK & APPETIZERS

Cucumber and Greek Yogurt Dip

Prep Time: 10 minutes Servings: 4

Ingredients:
- 1 cucumber, finely grated
- 1 cup low-fat Greek yogurt
- 2 cloves garlic, minced
- 1 tbsp fresh dill, cut
- Salt and pepper to taste

Directions:
1. Put the finely grated cucumber in a fine-mesh sieve and draw out excess liquid.
2. In a basin, mix together the grated cucumber, chopped dill, minced garlic, pepper, Greek yogurt, and salt.
3. Blend well until well mixed.
4. Refrigerate it for 30 minutes before serving.

Nutritional Information (per serving):
Calories: 40 Protein: 4g Sodium: 25mg Fiber: 1g Potassium: 200mg Phosphorus: 40mg Carbs: 5g

Baked Sweet Potato Fries

Prep Time: 15 minutes Cook Time: 25 minutes Servings: 4

Ingredients:
- 2 sweet potatoes, cut into fries
- 1 tbsp olive oil
- 1/2 tbsp paprika
- 1/2 tbsp garlic powder

- Salt and pepper to taste

Directions:

1. Set the oven temperature to 425°F (220°C).
2. In a basin, combine sweet potato fries with garlic powder, paprika, salt, olive oil, and pepper.
3. Arrange the fries on a baking sheet in a single layer.
4. Bake fries until they are crisp for 20 to 25 minutes, flipping once.
5. Serve hot.

Nutritional Information (per serving):

Calories: 120 Protein: 2g Sodium: 50mg Fiber: 3g Potassium: 400mg Phosphorus: 60mg Carbs: 24g

Caprese Skewers

Prep Time: 15 minutes Servings: 4

Ingredients:

- 16 cherry tomatoes
- 8 fresh mozzarella balls
- 16 fresh basil leaves
- 1 tbsp balsamic vinegar
- 1 tbsp olive oil
- Salt and pepper to taste

Directions:

1. Thread a mozzarella ball, cherry tomato, and a fresh basil leaf onto each skewer.
2. Organize the skewers on a platter.
3. Combine balsamic vinegar, olive oil, salt, and pepper in a small bowl.
4. Sprinkle the dressing over the skewers before serving.

Nutritional Information (per serving):

Calories: 120 Protein: 6g Sodium: 90mg Fiber: 1g Potassium: 240mg Phosphorus: 100mg Carbs: 2g

Avocado and Tomato Salsa

Prep Time: 10 minutes Servings: 4

Ingredients:
- 2 ripe avocados, diced
- 2 tomatoes, diced
- 1/4 cup red onion, finely chopped
- 1/4 cup fresh cilantro, diced
- 1 lime, juiced
- Salt and pepper to taste

Directions:
1. Combine the diced avocados, tomatoes, red onion, cilantro, lime juice, salt, and pepper in a bowl.
2. Mix well to combine.
3. Serve with whole-grain crackers or vegetable sticks.

Nutritional Information (per serving):
Calories: 140 Protein: 2g Sodium: 5mg Fiber: 5g Potassium: 520mg Phosphorus: 50mg Carbs: 11g

Roasted Red Pepper Hummus

Prep Time: 10 minutes Cook Time: 20 minutes (for roasting peppers) Servings: 6

Ingredients:
- 1 can (15 oz) rinsed and drained low-sodium chickpeas,
- 2 roasted red peppers, peeled and seeded
- 2 cloves garlic, minced
- 2 tbsps tahini
- 2 tbsps lemon juice
- 1 tbsp olive oil
- 1/2 tbsp ground cumin
- Salt and pepper to taste

Directions:

1. In a food processor, combine minced garlic, lemon juice, chickpeas, olive oil, roasted red peppers, tahini, ground cumin, pepper, and salt.
2. Process until smooth and has a creamy texture.
3. Serve with whole-grain pita bread or vegetable sticks.

Nutritional Information (per serving):

Calories: 120 Protein: 4g Sodium: 40mg Fiber: 3g Potassium: 160mg Phosphorus: 70mg Carbs: 15g

Greek Salad Cups

Prep Time: 15 minutes Servings: 4

Ingredients:

- 2 cucumbers, peeled and cut into rounds
- 1 cup cherry tomatoes, halved
- 1/2 cup pitted and cut Kalamata olives
- 1/2 cup crumbled feta cheese
- 1/4 cup red onion, finely chopped
- 2 tbsps fresh parsley, cut
- 2 tbsps balsamic vinegar
- 1 tbsp olive oil
- Salt and pepper to taste

Directions:

1. In a dish, combine cucumber rounds, crumbled feta cheese, sliced Kalamata olives, finely chopped red onion, halved cherry tomatoes, and chopped fresh parsley.
2. In a different dish, mix together olive oil, salt, balsamic vinegar, and pepper.
3. Sprinkle the dressing over the salad blend and lob to combine.
4. For a classy presentation, serve the salad in cucumber cups.

Nutritional Information (per serving):
Calories: 120 Protein: 4g Sodium: 370mg Fiber: 2g Potassium: 320mg Phosphorus: 90mg Carbs: 8g

Spicy Edamame

Prep Time: 10 minutes Cook Time: 5 minutes Servings: 4

Ingredients:
- 2 cups frozen edamame (shelled)
- 1 tbsp olive oil
- 1 tbsp chili powder
- 1/2 tbsp garlic powder
- 1/2 tbsp paprika
- Salt to taste

Directions:
1. Prepare the frozen edamame as directed on the package, typically by boiling or steaming for 5 minutes.
2. Drain and pat the edamame to dry.
3. In a basin, combine the salt, paprika, chile powder, olive oil, and cooked edamame.
4. Serve as a spicy and protein-packed snack.

Nutritional Information (per serving):
Calories: 130 Protein: 10g Sodium: 5mg Fiber: 6g Potassium: 230mg Phosphorus: 130mg Carbs: 8g

Cottage Cheese Stuffed Cucumber Cups

Prep Time: 15 minutes Servings: 4

Ingredients:
- 2 cucumbers, peeled and cut into rounds
- 1 cup low-fat cottage cheese
- 1/2 cup cherry tomatoes, halved
- 1/4 cup fresh basil leaves, torn

- 1/4 cup balsamic glaze
- Salt and pepper to taste

Directions:

1. In a basin, combine properly the low-fat cottage cheese, fresh basil leaves with cherry tomatoes.
2. Season with pepper and salt.
3. Insert the cottage cheese mixture into the cucumber rounds.
4. Sprinkle balsamic glaze atop before serving.

Nutritional Information (per serving):

Calories: 100 Protein: 12g Sodium: 390mg Fiber: 1g Potassium: 330mg Phosphorus: 120mg Carbs: 8g

Deviled Eggs

Prep Time: 20 minutes Cook Time: 12 minutes Servings: 4

Ingredients:

- 4 large eggs
- 2 tbsps low-fat mayonnaise
- 1 tbsp Dijon mustard
- 1/2 tbsp white vinegar
- 1/4 tbsp paprika
- Salt and pepper to taste
- Fresh parsley for garnish (optional)

Directions:

1. Add water to a pot with the eggs. Set on high heat until boil.
2. Turn off the heat, cover, and allow the eggs to sit in hot water for 12 minutes.
3. Remove eggs from the boiling water and place them in an ice bath to chill.
4. Peel the eggs and slice them in half lengthwise. Take out the yolks and put them in a dish.
5. Mash yolks with Dijon mustard, low-fat mayonnaise, paprika, salt, white vinegar, and pepper until smooth.

6. Fill the egg white halves with the yolk mixture.
7. If preferred, garnish with fresh parsley.

Nutritional Information (per serving):

Calories: 80 Protein: 6g Sodium: 150mg Fiber: 0g Potassium: 70mg Phosphorus: 90mg Carbs: 1g

Tzatziki Cucumber Bites

Prep Time: 15 minutes Servings: 4

Ingredients:

- 2 cucumbers, cut into rounds
- 1 cup low-fat Greek yogurt
- 1/2 cucumber, finely grated
- 2 cloves garlic, minced
- 1 tbsp fresh dill, cut
- Salt and pepper to taste
- Cherry tomatoes and fresh mint leaves for garnish (discretionary)

Directions:

1. In a basin, mix properly the finely grated cucumber, chopped fresh dill, minced garlic, low-fat Greek yogurt, pepper and salt.
2. Arrange rounds of cucumber on a serving dish.
3. Add a dollop of the yogurt mixture to the top of each cucumber round.
4. For garnishing, use the cherry tomatoes and fresh mint leaves as desired.

Nutritional Information (per serving):

Calories: 40 Protein: 4g Sodium: 30mg Fiber: 1g Potassium: 220mg Phosphorus: 40mg Carbs: 6g

CHAPTER SEVEN

BEVERAGES RECIPES

Fresh Strawberry Smoothie

Prep Time: 5 minutes Servings: 2

Ingredients:
- 1 cup of freshly hulled and halved strawberries
- 1 cup low-fat plain yogurt
- 1/2 cup almond milk (unsweetened)
- 1 tbsp honey (optional)
- 1/2 tbsp vanilla extract
- Ice cubes (optional)

Directions:
1. Put in a blender the low-fat plain yogurt, vanilla extract, almond milk, fresh strawberries, honey (optional), and ice cubes (choice).
2. Blend until you have a smooth consistency.
3. Pour into glasses and serve immediately.

Nutritional Information (per serving):
Calories: 120 Protein: 5g Sodium: 70mg Fiber: 2g Potassium: 320mg Phosphorus: 150mg Carbs: 20g

Green Tea Lemonade

Prep Time: 5 minutes Cook Time: 5 minutes Servings: 2

Ingredients:
- 2 green tea bags
- 2 cups hot water
- 1/4 cup freshly squeezed lemon juice
- 2 tbsps honey (optional)

- Ice cubes

Directions:

1. Soak green tea bags in boiled water for about 3-5 minutes.
2. Take out the tea bags, then allow the tea to cool to room temperature.
3. Add honey (if using) and freshly squeezed lemon juice.
4. Refrigerate it for some moment.
5. Serve over ice cubes.

Nutritional Information (per serving):

Calories: 20 Protein: 0g Sodium: 10mg Fiber: 0g Potassium: 30mg Phosphorus: 10mg Carbs: 5g

Watermelon Mint Cooler

Prep Time: 10 minutes Servings: 4

Ingredients:

- 4 cups fresh watermelon chunks, seeded
- 1/4 cup fresh mint leaves
- 2 tbsps freshly squeezed lime juice
- 1 tbsp honey (optional)
- Ice cubes

Directions:

1. Put in a blender the fresh watermelon chunks, freshly squeezed lime juice, fresh mint leaves, honey (if desired), and ice cubes.
2. Blend until you have a smooth consistency.
3. Sieve into a pitcher using a fine-mesh filter.
4. Refrigerate before serving.

Nutritional Information (per serving):

Calories: 40 Protein: 1g Sodium: 2mg Fiber: 1g Potassium: 220mg Phosphorus: 20mg Carbs: 10g

Beetroot and Carrot Juice

Prep Time: 10 minutes Servings: 2

Ingredients:

- 2 medium beetroots, peeled and sliced
- 4 medium carrots, peeled and sliced
- 1 apple, cored and sliced
- 1/2 lemon, peeled and seeded

Directions:

1. In a juicer, put the lemon, chopped beetroots, apple and carrots.
2. Process and extract the juice.
3. Decant into glasses and serve immediately.

Nutritional Information (per serving):

Calories: 80 Protein: 2g Sodium: 90mg Fiber: 4g Potassium: 610mg Phosphorus: 60mg Carbs: 20g

Ginger Turmeric Tea

Prep Time: 5 minutes Cook Time: 10 minutes Servings: 2

Ingredients:

- 2 cups water
- 1-inch fresh ginger, peeled and sliced
- 1 tbsp ground turmeric
- 1 tbsp honey (optional)
- 1/2 lemon, juiced

Directions:

1. Pour water into a saucepan, heat, and bring to a boil.
2. Add the powdered turmeric and ginger slices. Simmer for about 5-10 minutes.
3. Take out from heat and drain the tea into mugs.
4. Add the honey and lemon juice, if desired.
5. Serve hot.

Nutritional Information (per serving):

Calories: 5 Protein: 0g Sodium: 5mg Fiber: 0g Potassium: 40mg Phosphorus: 10mg Carbs: 2g

Pineapple and Coconut Water Smoothie

Prep Time: 5 minutes Servings: 2

Ingredients:

- 2 cups fresh pineapple chunks
- 1 cup coconut water
- 1/2 cup low-fat coconut milk
- 1/2 banana
- Ice cubes (optional)

Directions:

1. In a blender, add the fresh pineapple chunks, banana, low-fat coconut milk, coconut water, and ice cubes (if preferred).
2. Blend to get a smooth consistency.
3. Pour into glasses and serve immediately.

Nutritional Information (per serving):

Calories: 110 Protein: 2g Sodium: 75mg Fiber: 2g Potassium: 350mg Phosphorus: 60mg Carbs: 26g

Cucumber and Mint Infused Water

Prep Time: 5 minutes Servings: 2

Ingredients:

- 1 cucumber, thinly sliced
- 10 fresh mint leaves
- 4 cups water
- Ice cubes

Directions:

1. Combine fresh mint leaves and cucumber slices in a pitcher.
2. Add ice cubes and water.

3. Chill in the refrigerator for a few hours to let the flavors meld.
4. Serve chilled.

Nutritional Information (per serving):
Calories: 0 Protein: 0g Sodium: 0mg Fiber: 0g Potassium: 90mg Phosphorus: 10mg Carbs: 0g

Berry Blast Smoothie

Prep Time: 5 minutes Servings: 2

Ingredients:
- 1 cup assorted berries (raspberries, strawberries, blueberries)
- 1 cup low-fat plain yogurt
- 1/2 banana
- 1 tbsp honey (optional)
- Ice cubes (optional)

Directions:
1. In a blender, put the mixed berries, banana, low-fat plain yogurt, honey (optional), and ice cubes (if preferred).
2. Blend to get a smooth consistency.
3. Pour into glasses and serve immediately.

Nutritional Information (per serving):
Calories: 110 Protein: 5g Sodium: 60mg Fiber: 3g Potassium: 270mg Phosphorus: 160mg Carbs: 25g

Citrus Sunrise Smoothie

Prep Time: 5 minutes Servings: 2

Ingredients:
- 1 orange, peeled and segmented
- 1 grapefruit, peeled and segmented
- 1/2 cup low-fat plain yogurt
- 1 tbsp honey (optional)

- Ice cubes (optional)

Directions:

1. In a blender, put the grapefruit and orange segments, low-fat plain yogurt, honey (optional), and ice cubes (if preferred).
2. Blend to get a smooth consistency.
3. Pour into glasses and serve immediately.

Nutritional Information (per serving):

Calories: 120 Protein: 5g Sodium: 50mg Fiber: 3g Potassium: 450mg Phosphorus: 130mg Carbs: 26g

Iced Herbal Tea

Prep Time: 5 minutes Cook Time: 5 minutes Servings: 2

Ingredients:

- 2 herbal tea bags (e.g., chamomile, peppermint)
- 2 cups hot water
- 1 tbsp honey (optional)
- Ice cubes

Directions:

1. Soak herbal tea bags in boiled water for about 3-5 minutes.
2. Take out the tea bags, then allow the tea to cool to room temperature.
3. Add honey if desired.
4. Chill in the refrigerator.
5. Serve over ice cubes.

Nutritional Information (per serving):

Calories: 10 Protein: 0g Sodium: 5mg Fiber: 0g Potassium: 10mg Phosphorus: 10mg Carbs: 3g

CHAPTER EIGHT

MANAGING STRESS AND EXERCISE TIPS FOR STAGE 3 CKD

How Stress Affects Kidney Health

Stress can have a major negative influence on kidney function, particularly in people with Stage 3 Chronic Kidney Disease (CKD). The "fight-or-flight" response, often known as the stress response, causes a series of physiological changes while you are under stress. The following are some effects of stress on the kidneys and general health:

1. **Elevated Blood Pressure:** Stress chemicals like cortisol and adrenaline can cause elevated blood pressure. Increased blood pressure puts the kidneys under greater stress, which may eventually compromise renal function.

2. **Inflammation:** prolonged stress may result in systemic inflammation, which may harm renal blood vessels and compromise kidney function.

3. **Blood Sugar Fluctuations:** Stress can cause blood sugar levels to fluctuate, which is bad for those with CKD because irregular blood sugar levels can worsen renal damage.

4. **Immune System Suppression:** Chronic stress can impair immunity, leaving you more prone to infections. When the immune system is weak, kidney health may be jeopardized.

5. **Poor lifestyle choices: People** who are under a lot of stress may turn to unhealthy coping techniques including poor eating habits, drinking too much alcohol or caffeine, or cutting back on their physical activity. All of these actions can have a detrimental impact on kidney health.

The Value of Rest in Maintaining Kidney Health

In order to manage Stage 3 CKD and lessen the effects of stress on renal function, rest is essential. Getting enough rest and sleeping adequately is beneficial to your overall wellbeing:

1. **Blood Pressure Control:** Getting enough sleep is important for controlling blood pressure, which relieves kidney stress.

2. **Reduction of Inflammation:** Sleep allows the body to heal and rejuvenate, which helps to lower inflammation, a factor that can be harmful to renal function.

3. **Stress Reduction:** Getting enough restorative sleep increases one's ability to withstand stress, which lessens the damaging effects of stress on kidney health and makes it easier to deal with life's obstacles.

4. **Hormone Balance:** Sleep is crucial for maintaining hormonal equilibrium, which keeps stress hormones in control and ensures that metabolic hormones, like insulin, are working properly.

5. **Cellular Repair:** The body repairs and detoxifies its cells while you're sleeping deeply, which can help your kidneys and your general health.

Strategies to Enhance Rest

Make sleep a priority. Have a target of sleeping for 7-9 hours every night. Create a relaxing sleeping environment and establish a nighttime ritual.

Stress Reduction Methods: To promote peaceful sleep, use stress-reduction techniques like progressive muscle relaxation, mindfulness meditation, or deep breathing exercises.

Limit Stimulants: Before going to bed, stay away from caffeine and electrical devices since they can disrupt your sleep.

Regular Exercise: Regular, moderate-intensity exercise can enhance sleep patterns, so incorporate it into your regimen.

Speak with Your Healthcare Professional: Consult your healthcare professional if you experience sleep disorders or disruptions for guidance and appropriate therapies.

Exercises for Stage 3 Kidney Disease

Regular physical exercise is crucial in managing Stage 3 CKD. Maintaining muscle strength, enhancing cardiovascular health, and fostering general well-being are all benefits of exercise to any individual with stage 3 kidney disease.

Here are the types of exercises for your kidney health:

1. **Cardiovascular exercises:** These activities speed up your heartbeat and strengthen your heart. Examples of these are; brisk walking, swimming, and cycling.

2. **Strength Training:** Exercises that maintain muscle mass and strength are referred to as strength or resistance training. For upper and lower body exercises, use light weights or resistance bands.

3. **Flexibility and stretching:** Exercises that increase flexibility also lower the risk of muscle stiffness. To improve joint mobility, incorporate simple stretches into your routine.

4. **Balance training:** Stability is improved and the danger of falling is decreased through balance exercises like tai chi or particular yoga poses.

5. **Breathing exercises:** Breathing exercises can enhance lung function while lowering stress and anxiety. Deep breathing exercises are something that can be helpful.

6. **Low-Impact Activities:** People with joint discomfort or mobility problems may find activities like stationary cycling or water aerobics to be suitable because they are easy on the joints.

21 DAYS MEAL PLAN

Day 1:

- **Breakfast:** Greek Yogurt Parfait **(p. 29)**

- **Lunch:** Quinoa and Black Bean Salad **(p. 37)**

- **Dinner:** Lemon Herb Grilled Chicken **(p. 44)**

- **Snack:** Cucumber and Greek Yogurt Dip **(p. 54)**

- **Beverage:** Fresh Strawberry Smoothie **(p. 62)**

Day 2:

- **Breakfast:** Banana Nut Oatmeal **(p. 30)**

- **Lunch:** Spinach and Mushroom Stuffed Chicken Breast **(p. 38)**

- **Dinner:** Baked Cod with Tomato-Basil Sauce **(p. 45)**

- **Snack:** Baked Sweet Potato Fries **(p. 54)**

- **Beverage:** Green Tea Lemonade**(p. 62)**

Day 3:

- **Breakfast:** Avocado Toast with Poached Egg **(p. 32)**

- **Lunch:** Lentil and Vegetable Soup **(p. 39)**

- **Dinner:** Vegetable and Chickpea Stir-Fry **(p. 45)**

- **Snack:** Caprese Skewers **(p. 55)**

- **Beverage:** Watermelon Mint Cooler **(p. 63)**

Day 4:

- **Breakfast:** Spinach and Feta Scramble **(p. 29)**

- **Lunch:** Turkey and Avocado Wrap **(p. 40)**

- **Dinner:** Quinoa and Vegetable Pilaf **(p. 46)**

- **Snack:** Avocado and Tomato Salsa **(p. 56)**

- **Beverage:** Beetroot and Carrot Juice **(p. 64)**

Day 5:

- **Breakfast:** Berry Protein Smoothie **(p. 32)**

- **Lunch:** Vegetable Stir-Fry **(p. 40)**

- **Dinner:** Turkey and Vegetable Skewers **(p. 47)**

- **Snack:** Roasted Red Pepper Hummus **(p. 56)**

- **Beverage:** Ginger Turmeric Tea **(p. 64)**

Day 6:

- **Breakfast:** Spinach and Tomato Breakfast Quesadilla **(p. 31)**

- **Lunch:** Baked Salmon with Lemon-Dill Sauce **(p. 41)**

- **Dinner:** Lentil and Vegetable Stir-Fry **(p. 48)**

- **Snack:** Greek Salad Cups **(p. 57)**

- **Beverage:** Pineapple and Coconut Water Smoothie **(p. 65)**

Day 7:

- **Breakfast:** Cottage Cheese Pancakes **(p. 34)**
- **Lunch:** Eggplant and Tomato Stew **(p. 42)**
- **Dinner:** Spinach and Mushroom Stuffed Bell Peppers **(p. 49)**
- **Snack:** Spicy Edamame **(p. 58)**
- **Beverage:** Cucumber and Mint Infused Water **(p. 65)**

Day 8:

- **Breakfast:** Peanut Butter Banana Smoothie Bowl **(p. 35)**
- **Lunch:** Veggie and Hummus Wrap **(p. 43)**
- **Dinner:** Pork Tenderloin with Roasted Vegetables **(p. 50)**
- **Snack:** Cottage Cheese Stuffed Cucumber Cups **(p. 58)**
- **Beverage:** Berry Blast Smoothie **(p. 66)**

Day 9:

- **Breakfast:** Vegetable Omelette **(p. 28)**
- **Lunch:** Lentil and Vegetable Stir-Fry **(p. 48)**
- **Dinner:** Turkey Meatballs with Zucchini Noodles **(p. 51)**
- **Snack:** Deviled Eggs **(p. 59)**
- **Beverage:** Citrus Sunrise Smoothie **(p. 66)**

Day 10:

- **Breakfast:** Greek Yogurt Parfait **(p. 29)**

- **Lunch:** Spinach and Mushroom Stuffed Bell Peppers **(p. 49)**

- **Dinner:** Veggie and Brown Rice Bowl **(p. 52)**

- **Snack:** Tzatziki Cucumber Bites **(p. 60)**

- **Beverage:** Iced Herbal Tea **(p. 67)**

Day 11:

- **Breakfast:** Banana Nut Oatmeal **(p. 30)**

- **Lunch:** Grilled Chicken and Vegetable Salad **(p. 36)**

- **Dinner:** Lemon Herb Grilled Chicken **(p. 44)**

- **Snack:** Cucumber and Greek Yogurt Dip **(p. 54)**

- **Beverage:** Fresh Strawberry Smoothie **(p. 62)**

Day 12:

- **Breakfast:** Avocado Toast with Poached Egg **(p. 32)**

- **Lunch:** Quinoa and Black Bean Salad **(p. 37)**

- **Dinner:** Baked Cod with Tomato-Basil Sauce **(p. 45)**

- **Snack:** Baked Sweet Potato Fries **(p. 54)**

- **Beverage:** Green Tea Lemonade **(p. 62)**

Day 13:

- **Breakfast:** Spinach and Feta Scramble **(p. 29)**

- **Lunch:** Lentil and Vegetable Soup **(p. 39)**

- **Dinner:** Vegetable and Chickpea Stir-Fry **(p. 45)**

- **Snack:** Caprese Skewers **(p. 55)**

- **Beverage:** Watermelon Mint Cooler **(p. 63)**

Day 14:

- **Breakfast:** Berry Protein Smoothie **(p. 32)**

- **Lunch:** Turkey and Avocado Wrap **(p. 40)**

- **Dinner:** Quinoa and Vegetable Pilaf **(p. 46)**

- **Snack:** Avocado and Tomato Salsa **(p. 56)**

- **Beverage:** Beetroot and Carrot Juice **(p. 64)**

Day 15:

- **Breakfast:** Spinach and Tomato Breakfast Quesadilla **(p. 31)**

- **Lunch:** Vegetable Stir-Fry **(p. 40)**

- **Dinner:** Turkey and Vegetable Skewers **(p. 47)**

- **Snack:** Roasted Red Pepper Hummus **(p. 56)**

- **Beverage:** Ginger Turmeric Tea **(p. 64)**

Day 16:

- **Breakfast:** Avocado Toast with Poached Egg **(p. 32)**

- **Lunch:** Baked Salmon with Lemon-Dill Sauce **(p. 41)**

- **Dinner:** Lentil and Vegetable Stir-Fry **(p. 48)**

- **Snack:** Greek Salad Cups **(p. 57**

- **Beverage:** Pineapple and Coconut Water Smoothie **(p. 65)**

Day 17:

- **Break Breakfast:** Cottage Cheese Pancakes **(p. 34)**

- **Lunch:** Eggplant and Tomato Stew **(p. 42)**

- **Dinner:** Spinach and Mushroom Stuffed Bell Peppers **(p. 49)**

- **Snack:** Spicy Edamame **(p. 58)**

- **Beverage:** Cucumber and Mint Infused Water **(p. 65)**

Day 18:

- **Breakfast:** Peanut Butter Banana Smoothie Bowl **(p. 35)**

- **Lunch:** Veggie and Hummus Wrap **(p. 43)**

- **Dinner:** Pork Tenderloin with Roasted Vegetables **(p. 50)**

- **Snack:** Cottage Cheese Stuffed Cucumber Cups **(p. 58)**

- **Beverage:** Berry Blast Smoothie **(p. 66)**

Day 19:

- **Breakfast:** Vegetable Omelette **(p. 28)**

- **Lunch:** Lentil and Vegetable Stir-Fry **(p. 39)**

- **Dinner:** Turkey Meatballs with Zucchini Noodles **(p. 51)**

- **Snack:** Deviled Eggs **(p. 59)**

- **Beverage:** Citrus Sunrise Smoothie **(p. 66)**

Day 20:

- **Breakfast:** Greek Yogurt Parfait **(p. 29)**

- **Lunch:** Spinach and Mushroom Stuffed Bell Peppers **(p. 33)**

- **Dinner:** Veggie and Brown Rice Bowl **(p. 52)**

- **Snack:** Tzatziki Cucumber Bites **(p. 60)**

- **Beverage:** Iced Herbal Tea **(p. 67)**

Day 21:

- **Breakfast:** Banana Nut Oatmeal **(p. 30)**

- **Lunch:** Grilled Chicken and Vegetable Salad **(p. 36)**

- **Dinner:** Lemon Herb Grilled Chicken **(p. 44)**

- **Snack:** Cucumber and Greek Yogurt Dip **(p. 54)**

- **Beverage:** Fresh Strawberry Smoothie **(p. 62)**

14-DAY EXERCISE PLAN

This 14-day fitness program is specifically designed for people with Stage 3 Chronic Kidney Disease (CKD). The low-impact activities that are the emphasis of this plan gradually becoming more intense. Never begin an exercise program without first talking to your doctor or nephrologist.

Day 1 – 3: Gentle Cardiovascular Exercise

- **Day 1:** Get started with a 10-minute walk at a pace you deem comfortable.
- **Day 2:** Extend your walk to 15 minutes.
- **Day 3:** Add an extra 5, making it 20 minutes.

Day 4-6: Strength and Flexibility Training

- Day 4: Start with a 5-minute light flexibility stretches, then add 5 minutes of gentle resistance band exercises.
- Day 5: Extend both exercises to 10 minutes apiece.
- Day 6: Intensify the stretching and resistance exercises to 15 minutes each.
- Day 7: Take a break and rest to recover

Day 8-10: Cardio and Balance Training

- **Day 8:** Restart a 20-minute walk.

- **Day 9:** After your walk, perform balancing drills like standing on one leg for 30 seconds at a time.
- **Day 10:** Extend your walk to 25 minutes and keep up your balancing drills.

Day 11-13: Strength and Flexibility Training

- **Day 11:** Restart stretching and resistance exercises for 15 minutes each.
- **Day 12:** Intensify the timing of the exercises to 20 minutes apiece.
- **Day 13:** Perform 25 minutes of both stretching and resistance exercises.

Day 14: Rest and Recovery

Take a day off to relax and give your body time to heal.

Don't forget to drink plenty of water and pay attention to your body during this 14-day fitness program. Adjust the exercises as necessary if you feel any pain or discomfort, or speak with your healthcare provider.

Depending on your development and comfort level, you might choose to repeat or change this two-week plan after finishing it. Your general fitness can be enhanced and your kidney health can be supported by gradually increasing the time and intensity of your workouts. Always put safety first, and when looking for personalized fitness advice, talk to your medical team.

CONCLUSION

As **Kidney Disease Diet Cookbook For Stage 3** draws to a close, let's take a moment to consider the incredible adventure we've been on. We looked into the complex realm of Stage 3 Chronic Kidney Disease (CKD), its causes, symptoms, and the crucial value of early treatments. We have uncovered the critical function that diet plays in maintaining kidney health, mastered the skill of developing kidney-friendly meal plans, and unraveled the secrets of essential nutrients. With smart shopping strategies and meal prep hacks, we have successfully navigated the challenges of managing salt, potassium, and phosphorus. We've started a culinary journey where we learned how to make nutrient-rich breakfast, lunch, supper, snack, and beverage recipes that are good for the body and the soul.

But this is not where our journey ends. It permeates more than just these pages; it affects your life, daily decisions, and kitchen. It is a path characterized by empowerment, transformation, and the firm conviction that you have the ability to positively impact the health of your kidneys.

More than just the discovery of a plethora of recipes, you have also found hope. The hope that, with each meal you cook, each grocery list you make, and each mouthful you relish, you're making progress toward a healthier, more fulfilling future. You have embraced the fact that exercise helps build stronger kidneys in addition to improving physical well-being. You have also understood the serious impacts that stress may have on the health of your kidneys and the significance of rest in your recovery.

As you proceed, keep in mind that your journey is unique to you. Although your experience is unique, it is connected with the stories of millions of others who have suffered or are currently confronting the difficulties of kidney disease. Your loved ones, your healthcare team, and the knowledge in these pages will all be there to assist you as you travel this route.

What lies ahead then? A 14-day workout program created with your well-being in mind, a 21-day eating plan to jump-start your kidney-healthy lifestyle, and the knowledge that you now have the resources to significantly improve your kidney health.

Finally, keep in mind that this book is only one chapter of your health's continuous story. As you close this guide and kick-start your journey, remember you have the ability to shape your story. Let it be a story about tenacity, about hope, and about the amazing power of the human spirit.

Thank you once again for choosing the **Kidney Disease Diet Cookbook for Stage 3** as your guide on this journey. I am committed to helping you achieve your health goals and improve your quality of life.

If you found this book helpful, I would greatly appreciate it if you could leave a positive review. Your review will help others who are looking for a guide to manage their chronic kidney disease.

Thank you again for your support.

ACCESS TO MY OTHER BOOKS

I have other books that you could find helpful. Kindly scan the code below to gain access.

OR

https://www.amazon.com/author/michgreen

BONUS

WEEKLY MEAL PLANNER

Weekly Meal Planner

Date: _____

	BREAKFAST	LUNCH	DINNER	SNACKS
MON				
TUE				
WED				
THU				
FRI				
SAT				
SUN				

SHOPPING LIST

- _____
- _____
- _____
- _____
- _____
- _____
- _____
- _____

NOTES

○
○
○
○
○
○

Weekly Meal Planner

Date: _____

	BREAKFAST	LUNCH	DINNER	SNACKS
MON				
TUE				
WED				
THU				
FRI				
SAT				
SUN				

SHOPPING LIST

- _____
- _____
- _____
- _____
- _____
- _____
- _____
- _____

NOTES

○
○
○
○
○

Weekly Meal Planner

Date: _____

	BREAKFAST	LUNCH	DINNER	SNACKS
MON				
TUE				
WED				
THU				
FRI				
SAT				
SUN				

SHOPPING LIST

- _____
- _____
- _____
- _____
- _____
- _____
- _____
- _____

NOTES

○
○
○
○
○

Weekly Meal Planner

Date: _____

	BREAKFAST	LUNCH	DINNER	SNACKS
MON				
TUE				
WED				
THU				
FRI				
SAT				
SUN				

SHOPPING LIST

- _____
- _____
- _____
- _____
- _____
- _____
- _____
- _____

NOTES

○

○

○

○

○

Weekly Meal Planner

Date: _____

	BREAKFAST	LUNCH	DINNER	SNACKS
MON				
TUE				
WED				
THU				
FRI				
SAT				
SUN				

SHOPPING LIST

- _____
- _____
- _____
- _____
- _____
- _____
- _____
- _____

NOTES

○
○
○
○
○

Weekly Meal Planner

Date: _____

	BREAKFAST	LUNCH	DINNER	SNACKS
MON				
TUE				
WED				
THU				
FRI				
SAT				
SUN				

SHOPPING LIST

- _____
- _____
- _____
- _____
- _____
- _____
- _____
- _____

NOTES

Weekly Meal Planner

Date: _____

	BREAKFAST	LUNCH	DINNER	SNACKS
MON				
TUE				
WED				
THU				
FRI				
SAT				
SUN				

SHOPPING LIST

- _____
- _____
- _____
- _____
- _____
- _____
- _____
- _____

NOTES

○
○
○
○
○
○

Weekly Meal Planner

Date: _____

	BREAKFAST	LUNCH	DINNER	SNACKS
MON				
TUE				
WED				
THU				
FRI				
SAT				
SUN				

SHOPPING LIST

- _____
- _____
- _____
- _____
- _____
- _____
- _____
- _____

NOTES

○
○
○
○
○

Weekly Meal Planner

Date: _____

	BREAKFAST	LUNCH	DINNER	SNACKS
MON				
TUE				
WED				
THU				
FRI				
SAT				
SUN				

SHOPPING LIST

- _____
- _____
- _____
- _____
- _____
- _____
- _____
- _____

NOTES

○
○
○
○
○

Weekly Meal Planner

Date: _____

	BREAKFAST	LUNCH	DINNER	SNACKS
MON				
TUE				
WED				
THU				
FRI				
SAT				
SUN				

SHOPPING LIST

- _____
- _____
- _____
- _____
- _____
- _____
- _____
- _____

NOTES

○
○
○
○
○

Made in the USA
Coppell, TX
28 June 2024

34047312R00056